COMPREHENSIVE GUIDE TO LIVING WITH TINNITUS

Tools, Tips, and Techniques for Finding Relief and Managing Ringing Ears

LOUIS LANHAM

Copyright © 2024 by Louis Lanham

All rights reserved. No part of this publication may be reproduced, stored, or transmitted in any form or by any means, electronic, mechanical, photocopying, recording, scanning, or otherwise, without written permission from the publisher. It is illegal to copy this book, post it to a website, or distribute it by any other means without permission

TABLE OF CONTENTS

INTRODUCTION

What is Tinnitus?

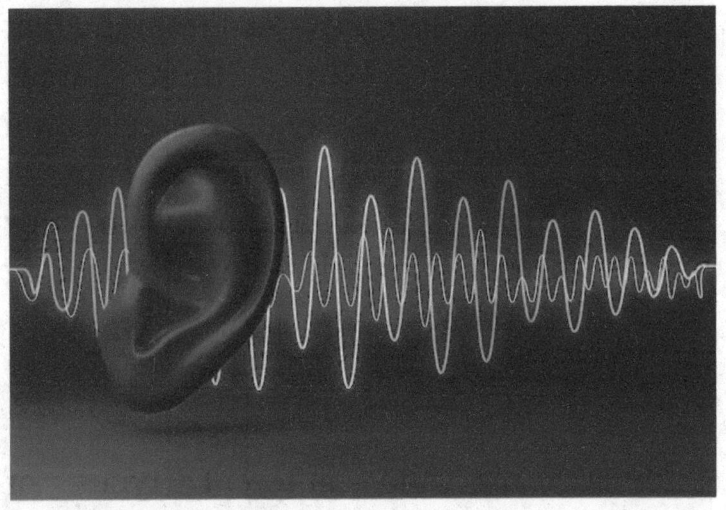

Tinnitus is a condition where a person hears sounds that aren't coming from an external source. It's often described as "ringing in the ears," but it can also sound like buzzing, hissing, whistling, or clicking. For some people, these sounds are a minor nuisance, while for others, they can be overwhelming and affect daily life.

Tinnitus is not a disease itself but a symptom of an underlying condition. It occurs when there's a problem in the auditory system, which includes the ear, the auditory nerve, and parts of the brain that process sound. When these areas malfunction, they can create the sensation of sound even when there is none. Think of it like an electrical short circuit in your brain's wiring that tricks you into hearing something that isn't there.

Types of Tinnitus

Understanding the different types of tinnitus can help in diagnosing and treating the condition effectively. Here are the main types:

→ **Subjective Tinnitus**:
  ◆ **Description**: This is the most common type of tinnitus. Only the person experiencing it can hear the sounds.

- ◆ **Causes**: It's often caused by problems in the inner ear or auditory nerve and can be triggered by factors like exposure to loud noises, ear infections, or age-related hearing loss.

→ **Objective Tinnitus**:
- ◆ **Description**: This type is rare and can be heard by both the person experiencing it and others, such as a doctor during an examination.
- ◆ **Causes**: It's usually due to a physical issue, such as a blood vessel problem, muscle contractions, or a middle ear bone condition. Because it has a clear physical source, it's sometimes easier to treat.

→ **Somatic Tinnitus**:
- ◆ **Description**: This type is associated with movement. The sounds can change or be

influenced by physical actions, such as turning the head, clenching the jaw, or moving the neck.

- ◆ **Causes**: It's often related to muscle spasms or issues with the neck or jaw, like temporomandibular joint (TMJ) disorder.

→ **Pulsatile Tinnitus**:

- ◆ **Description**: With pulsatile tinnitus, the sound pulses in rhythm with your heartbeat. This type of tinnitus can be particularly distressing because of its rhythmic nature.
- ◆ **Causes**: It's typically linked to changes in blood flow or blood vessels near the ears. Conditions such as high blood pressure, anemia, or an aneurysm can cause pulsatile tinnitus.

By understanding these types, we can better grasp the complexities of tinnitus and the various ways it can manifest. This knowledge is crucial for finding the right treatment and coping strategies to improve the quality of life for those affected by this condition.

Prevalence and Impact

Statistics

Tinnitus is a common condition that affects millions of people worldwide. According to recent studies:

- Approximately 10-15% of the global population experiences some form of tinnitus.
- In the United States, around 50 million people report experiencing tinnitus, with about 20 million suffering from chronic tinnitus and 2 million experiencing severe, debilitating cases.
- Tinnitus is more prevalent in older adults, particularly those over 60, but

it can affect people of all ages, including children.

These statistics highlight the widespread nature of tinnitus and underscore the importance of understanding and addressing this condition.

How Tinnitus Affects Daily Life

The impact of tinnitus on daily life can vary greatly from person to person. For some, it is a minor annoyance, while for others, it can be a significant source of distress and discomfort. Here are some ways tinnitus can affect individuals:

- **Sleep Disturbances**: Many people with tinnitus have trouble falling asleep or staying asleep due to the constant noise in their ears. This can lead to chronic sleep deprivation and associated health problems.
- **Concentration and Focus**: The persistent sound can make it difficult

to concentrate on tasks, whether at work, school, or home. This can affect productivity and performance.

- **Emotional Well-being**: Tinnitus can cause feelings of frustration, anxiety, and depression. The constant noise can be overwhelming, leading to a sense of helplessness and decreased quality of life.
- **Social Interactions**: People with severe tinnitus may avoid social situations because of difficulty hearing conversations over the internal noise or because they feel self-conscious about their condition. This can lead to social isolation.
- **Hearing Loss**: Tinnitus is often associated with hearing loss, which can further complicate communication and exacerbate the condition's impact on daily life.

What Readers Will Learn

This book aims to provide comprehensive information and practical guidance for those affected by tinnitus, as well as for their families, friends, and healthcare providers. Here's what readers can expect to learn:

1. **Understanding Tinnitus**: Readers will gain a clear understanding of what tinnitus is, including its causes, types, and how it affects the auditory system.

2. **Identifying Symptoms and Seeking Diagnosis**: The book will help readers recognize the symptoms of tinnitus and understand the diagnostic process, including when and how to seek medical advice.

3. **Exploring Treatment Options**: A detailed look at the various treatment options available, both medical and alternative, to help manage and alleviate tinnitus symptoms.

4. **Coping Strategies**: Practical tips and strategies for managing the impact of tinnitus on daily life, including techniques for reducing

stress and improving sleep and concentration.

5. **Lifestyle Adjustments**: Advice on lifestyle changes that can help minimize the effects of tinnitus, such as dietary adjustments, exercise, and sound therapy.

6. **Technological Advances**: An overview of the latest advancements in tinnitus research and treatment, providing hope for future relief and potential cures.

7. **Resources and Support**: Information on where to find additional help and support, including organizations, support groups, and online communities.

By providing this knowledge, the book aims to empower readers to take control of their tinnitus, improve their quality of life, and find support and relief in their journey.

CHAPTER 1:

The Science Behind Tinnitus

The Auditory System

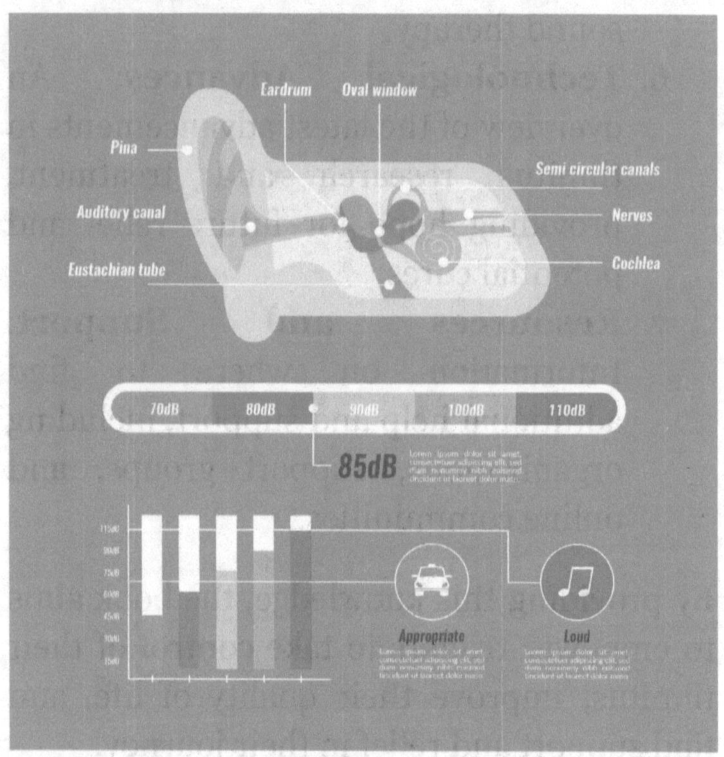

How Hearing Works

Hearing is a complex process that involves several steps, converting sound waves into electrical signals that the brain can interpret. Here's a simplified overview:

1. **Sound Wave Collection**: Sound waves enter the ear through the outer ear (pinna) and travel down the ear canal.
2. **Eardrum Vibration**: These sound waves hit the eardrum (tympanic membrane), causing it to vibrate.
3. **Middle Ear Bones**: The vibrations from the eardrum are transmitted to the three tiny bones in the middle ear (ossicles: malleus, incus, and stapes). These bones amplify the vibrations and pass them to the inner ear.
4. **Cochlea Activation**: In the inner ear, the vibrations reach the cochlea, a spiral-shaped organ filled with fluid. The movement of the fluid stimulates tiny hair cells lining the cochlea.

5. **Electrical Signal Generation**: The hair cells convert the mechanical vibrations into electrical signals.

6. **Signal Transmission**: These electrical signals travel along the auditory nerve to the brain, where they are interpreted as sound.

Anatomy of the Ear

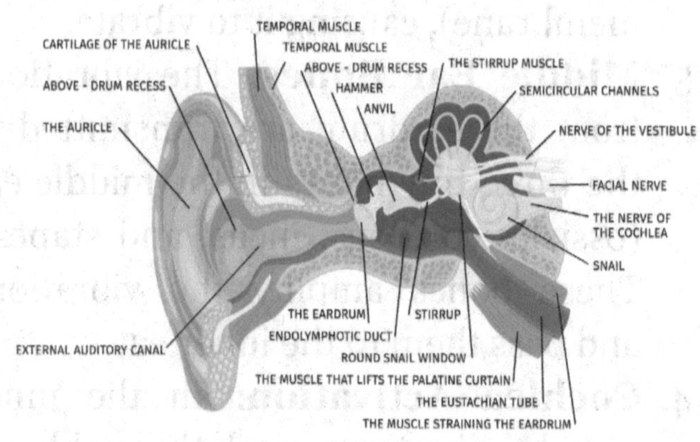

Understanding the anatomy of the ear helps in grasping how hearing works and how tinnitus can develop. The ear is divided into three main parts:

1.Outer Ear:

- **Pinna (Auricle)**: The visible part of the ear that collects sound waves.
- **Ear Canal**: The passage leading to the eardrum.
- **Eardrum (Tympanic Membrane)**: A thin membrane that vibrates when sound waves hit it.

2. Middle Ear:

- **Ossicles**: The three small bones (malleus, incus, stapes) that amplify sound vibrations.
- **Eustachian Tube**: Connects the middle ear to the back of the nose and helps equalize pressure.

3. Inner Ear:

- **Cochlea**: A fluid-filled, spiral-shaped structure that contains hair cells which convert vibrations into electrical signals.

- **Semicircular Canals**: Part of the balance system, not directly involved in hearing.
- **Auditory Nerve**: Carries electrical signals from the cochlea to the brain.

Mechanisms of Tinnitus

Neural Pathways

Tinnitus involves complex neural pathways that include the auditory system and parts of the brain responsible for processing sound. Below is how these pathways work:

1. **Signal Transmission**: Sound information is transmitted from the cochlea through the auditory nerve to the brainstem.
2. **Brainstem Processing**: The brainstem plays a crucial role in sound localization and reflexive responses to sound.

3. **Thalamus Relay**: Sound signals are relayed through the thalamus, which acts as a hub for sensory information.

4. **Cortex Interpretation**: The primary auditory cortex in the brain processes these signals, interpreting them as recognizable sounds.

The Brain's Role in Tinnitus

Tinnitus is not just an ear problem; it involves how the brain interprets and processes sound. Here are some key points about the brain's role in tinnitus:

1.Abnormal Neural Activity: In tinnitus, the brain may misinterpret normal neural activity as sound. This can happen due to damage or changes in the auditory system.

2. Hyperactivity and Reorganization: When the brain receives less input from the ears (due to hearing loss or damage), it can become hyperactive or reorganize itself, leading to the perception of sound (tinnitus).

3. Emotional Response: The limbic system, which controls emotions, can become involved. This is why tinnitus can be distressing and why stress or anxiety can worsen it.

4. Feedback Loops: Persistent tinnitus can create feedback loops in the brain, reinforcing the perception of sound and making it more difficult to ignore.

Understanding these mechanisms helps in identifying potential targets for treatment and management of tinnitus, highlighting the importance of both the ear and the brain in this condition.

Causes of Tinnitus

Tinnitus can be caused by various underlying factors, some more common than others. Understanding these causes can help in both preventing and treating the condition. Here are the main causes:

Hearing Loss

One of the most common causes of tinnitus is hearing loss, which often comes with age or from prolonged exposure to loud noises.

- **Age-Related Hearing Loss (Presbycusis)**: As people age, the delicate hair cells in the cochlea can degrade, leading to hearing loss and often tinnitus. This type of hearing loss typically starts around age 60 and progresses over time.
- **Noise-Induced Hearing Loss**: Exposure to loud noises, whether from occupational settings (e.g., construction, music industry) or recreational activities (e.g., concerts, loud music), can damage the hair cells in the inner ear. Once these cells are damaged, they cannot be repaired, leading to permanent hearing loss and often tinnitus.

Ear Infections

Ear infections can cause temporary tinnitus by affecting the middle or inner ear.

- **Middle Ear Infections (Otitis Media)**: These infections cause fluid buildup and inflammation in the middle ear, which can affect hearing and lead to temporary tinnitus.
- **Inner Ear Infections (Labyrinthitis)**: Infections that affect the inner ear can lead to inflammation and damage to the auditory pathways, potentially causing tinnitus.

Noise Exposure

Acute or chronic exposure to loud noises is a significant cause of tinnitus.

- **Acute Noise Trauma**: Sudden exposure to extremely loud noises, such as explosions or gunshots, can cause immediate hearing damage and result in tinnitus.

- **Chronic Noise Exposure**: Long-term exposure to high noise levels, such as those experienced in certain workplaces or through the use of headphones at high volumes, can lead to gradual hearing loss and tinnitus.

Other Medical Conditions

Several medical conditions can cause or contribute to tinnitus. Some of these include:

- **Earwax Blockage**: Excessive earwax can block the ear canal, causing pressure and affecting the eardrum's function, leading to tinnitus. Removing the earwax can often relieve the symptoms.
- **Ménière's Disease**: This inner ear disorder is characterized by episodes of vertigo, hearing loss, and tinnitus.

The exact cause is unknown, but it involves abnormal fluid pressure in the inner ear.

- **Otosclerosis**: This hereditary condition causes abnormal bone growth in the middle ear, affecting the ossicles' ability to transmit sound. It can lead to hearing loss and tinnitus.

- **Head and Neck Injuries**: Trauma to the head or neck can impact the auditory nerves or the brain's hearing centers, resulting in tinnitus.

- **Cardiovascular Conditions**: Conditions like high blood pressure, atherosclerosis, or abnormal blood flow can cause pulsatile tinnitus, where the tinnitus pulses in sync with the heartbeat.

- **Temporomandibular Joint (TMJ) Disorders**: Issues with the TMJ, which connects the jaw to the skull, can cause tinnitus due to the proximity of the joint to the ear.

- **Medications**: Certain medications, such as high doses of aspirin, antibiotics, or diuretics, can cause tinnitus as a side effect. This type of tinnitus is usually reversible once the medication is stopped.
- **Chronic Health Conditions**: Conditions such as diabetes, thyroid problems, and autoimmune diseases can also contribute to tinnitus.

Identifying the specific cause of tinnitus in an individual can be challenging, as it may result from multiple factors. However, understanding these causes is essential for developing effective treatment and management strategies.

CHAPTER 2:

Symptoms and Diagnosis

Common Sounds and Sensations

Tinnitus manifests in various sounds and sensations that can differ from person to person. These sounds can be constant or intermittent and may vary in pitch and volume. Common descriptions of tinnitus sounds include:

- **Ringing**: A high-pitched sound similar to a bell or telephone.
- **Buzzing**: A continuous, low-pitched sound like a buzzing bee.
- **Hissing**: A sound similar to steam escaping or white noise.
- **Whistling**: A high-pitched, whistling tone.
- **Clicking**: Rhythmic clicking noises, which may come and go.
- **Roaring**: A sound like ocean waves or a roaring engine.

- **Whooshing**: A pulsing noise that often coincides with the heartbeat, known as pulsatile tinnitus.

These sounds can be heard in one ear (unilateral tinnitus) or both ears (bilateral tinnitus) and may also seem to come from inside the head.

Severity and Frequency

The severity and frequency of tinnitus can vary widely among individuals. Factors that influence these variations include the underlying cause, overall health, and exposure to triggers such as loud noises or stress. Tinnitus can be classified based on its impact on daily life:

- **Mild Tinnitus**: This form is often an occasional nuisance and can be easily ignored or masked by environmental sounds. It typically does not interfere significantly with daily activities.

- **Moderate Tinnitus**: This form is more persistent and can cause noticeable discomfort. It may interfere with concentration and sleep, but individuals can generally manage it with coping strategies and treatments.
- **Severe Tinnitus**: This form is constant and can be debilitating. It significantly affects the quality of life, making it difficult to concentrate, sleep, and engage in social activities. Severe tinnitus often requires comprehensive treatment and support.

When to See a Doctor

Tinnitus can be a sign of an underlying health issue, so it's essential to know when to seek medical advice. Here are some guidelines:

- **Persistent Tinnitus**: If you experience tinnitus for more than a few days, it's a good idea to see a doctor, especially if it's bothersome or worsening.

- **Sudden Onset**: If tinnitus comes on suddenly, particularly if it's in one ear or accompanied by hearing loss, dizziness, or balance issues, seek immediate medical attention.
- **Significant Impact on Daily Life**: If tinnitus interferes with your ability to sleep, concentrate, or perform daily activities, a healthcare provider can help identify coping strategies and treatments.
- **Associated Symptoms**: If tinnitus is accompanied by other symptoms such as ear pain, drainage, or vertigo, it could indicate an ear infection or another condition that requires medical intervention.

Diagnostic Tests

To diagnose the cause of tinnitus, a healthcare provider will perform several tests. These may include:

1.Medical History and Physical Examination:

- **History**: The doctor will ask about your medical history, lifestyle, and the specifics of your tinnitus, such as the onset, duration, and characteristics of the sounds you hear.
- **Physical Exam**: A thorough examination of the ears, head, and neck to check for any obvious issues, such as earwax blockage or ear infections.

2. Hearing Tests:

- **Pure Tone Audiometry**: Measures your hearing sensitivity at different frequencies to detect hearing loss, which is often associated with tinnitus.
- **Speech Audiometry**: Evaluates your ability to hear and understand speech, which can be affected by hearing loss.

- **Tympanometry**: Assesses the function of the middle ear and eardrum, checking for fluid, ear infections, or eustachian tube dysfunction.

3. Imaging Tests:

- **Magnetic Resonance Imaging (MRI)**: Used to rule out tumors or other abnormalities in the auditory nerve and brain.
- **Computed Tomography (CT) Scan**: Helps detect structural problems in the ear and surrounding areas.

4. Additional Tests:

- **Blood Tests**: To identify underlying health conditions such as thyroid problems, anemia, or diabetes that could contribute to tinnitus.
- **Balance Tests**: If tinnitus is accompanied by dizziness or balance issues, tests like

electronystagmography (ENG) or videonystagmography (VNG) can assess the vestibular system.

Differential Diagnosis

Tinnitus can be a symptom of many different conditions, so differentiating it from other potential causes is crucial for accurate diagnosis and treatment. Here are some conditions that may be considered in the differential diagnosis:

1.**Ménière's Disease**: Characterized by tinnitus, fluctuating hearing loss, vertigo, and a feeling of fullness in the ear. It typically affects one ear and can cause episodic attacks.

2. **Acoustic Neuroma (Vestibular Schwannoma)**: A benign tumor on the auditory nerve that can cause unilateral tinnitus, hearing loss, and balance issues. MRI is often used to diagnose this condition.

3. Temporomandibular Joint (TMJ) Disorders: Problems with the jaw joint can cause tinnitus, jaw pain, headaches, and clicking sounds when moving the jaw. A dental or TMJ specialist may be involved in the diagnosis and treatment.

4. Eustachian Tube Dysfunction: Occurs when the eustachian tube, which equalizes pressure in the middle ear, doesn't function properly. Symptoms include a feeling of fullness in the ears, muffled hearing, and tinnitus.

5. Otosclerosis: A hereditary condition involving abnormal bone growth in the middle ear, leading to conductive hearing loss and tinnitus. Hearing tests and imaging may be used for diagnosis.

6. Vascular Disorders: Conditions such as high blood pressure, atherosclerosis, or arteriovenous malformations can cause pulsatile tinnitus. Vascular imaging studies may be required for diagnosis.

Accurate diagnosis through a combination of medical history, physical examination, and appropriate tests is essential for determining the underlying cause of tinnitus and developing an effective treatment plan.

CHAPTER 3:

Types of Tinnitus

Subjective Tinnitus

Subjective tinnitus is the most common form of tinnitus, accounting for more than 95% of cases. It is a condition where only the person affected can hear the sounds. These sounds are not generated by any external source, and no one else, including a doctor, can hear them through an examination. Here are the key aspects of subjective tinnitus:

Causes

1.Hearing Loss:

- **Age-Related Hearing Loss (Presbycusis):** As people age, the hair cells in the inner ear can deteriorate, leading to reduced hearing and tinnitus.

- **Noise-Induced Hearing Loss**: Exposure to loud noises, whether sudden or prolonged, can damage the hair cells in the cochlea, resulting in hearing loss and tinnitus.

2. Ear Infections and Blockages:

- **Middle Ear Infections (Otitis Media)**: Infections can cause fluid buildup and inflammation, which may lead to tinnitus.
- **Earwax Blockage**: Excessive earwax can block the ear canal, causing pressure changes and tinnitus. Removing the earwax often alleviates the symptoms.

3. Ototoxic Medications: Some medications can be toxic to the inner ear, leading to tinnitus. These include certain antibiotics, diuretics, chemotherapy drugs, and high doses of aspirin.

4. Head and Neck Injuries: Trauma to the head or neck can damage the auditory pathways or affect blood flow to the ears, causing tinnitus.

5. Chronic Health Conditions:

- **Hypertension**: High blood pressure can increase the risk of developing tinnitus.
- **Diabetes**: Poor blood sugar control can damage the auditory system, leading to tinnitus.
- **Thyroid Disorders**: Both hyperthyroidism and hypothyroidism can be associated with tinnitus.

6. Stress and Anxiety: Psychological factors such as stress and anxiety can exacerbate tinnitus symptoms. The exact mechanism is not well understood, but it is believed that stress can increase the brain's perception of tinnitus.

7. Meniere's Disease: This inner ear disorder causes episodes of vertigo, hearing loss, and tinnitus. It is associated with abnormal fluid pressure in the inner ear.

<u>Characteristics</u>

1.Perceived Sounds: The sounds experienced in subjective tinnitus can vary widely. Common descriptions include ringing, buzzing, hissing, clicking, and roaring. These sounds can be continuous or intermittent and may vary in pitch and volume.

2. Localization: Tinnitus can be perceived in one ear (unilateral) or both ears (bilateral). It can also feel like it is coming from inside the head.

3. Variability: The intensity and frequency of tinnitus can fluctuate. Some people may experience mild symptoms that are barely noticeable, while others may have severe symptoms that significantly affect their quality of life.

4. Impact on Daily Life: The impact of subjective tinnitus on daily life varies. It can cause sleep disturbances, difficulty concentrating, emotional distress, and social withdrawal. The severity of these effects often correlates with the loudness and persistence of the tinnitus sounds.

5. Associated Symptoms: In addition to the perceived sounds, people with subjective tinnitus may experience hearing loss, a feeling of fullness in the ears, and sensitivity to loud noises (hyperacusis).

Objective Tinnitus

Objective tinnitus is a rare form of tinnitus that can be heard by both the affected individual and an examiner using a stethoscope or other listening devices. Unlike subjective tinnitus, the sounds in objective tinnitus have a physical source within the body, often related to blood flow or muscle activity.

Causes

→ **Vascular Disorders**:
  ◆ **Arteriovenous Malformations (AVMs)**:

Abnormal connections between arteries and veins can create turbulent blood flow, leading to pulsatile tinnitus that can be heard by others.

◆ **Carotid Artery Stenosis**: Narrowing of the carotid artery can cause turbulent blood flow, producing a pulsating sound in the ear.

◆ **High Blood Pressure**: Elevated blood pressure can increase the force of blood flow, contributing to pulsatile tinnitus.

→ **Muscle Spasms**:

◆ **Middle Ear Myoclonus**: Involuntary muscle contractions in the middle ear muscles, such as the tensor tympani or stapedius muscles, can produce clicking or buzzing sounds that are audible to an examiner.

→ **Eustachian Tube Dysfunction**:

◆ **Patulous Eustachian Tube**:
When the eustachian tube
remains open, sounds of
breathing and internal bodily
noises can be transmitted to the
ear, resulting in objective
tinnitus.

→ **Glomus Tumors**:

◆ **Paragangliomas**: These
benign vascular tumors located
in the ear or near the base of the
skull can produce a pulsatile
tinnitus due to their blood flow
dynamics.

Characteristics

→ **Perceived Sounds**:

◆ The sounds in objective tinnitus
can include pulsatile noises,
clicking, or buzzing. These
sounds are typically rhythmic
and may coincide with the
heartbeat (pulsatile tinnitus) or
muscle contractions.

→ **Localization**:
  ◆ Objective tinnitus is often localized to one ear (unilateral), but in some cases, it can affect both ears (bilateral), depending on the source of the sound.

→ **Detectability**:
  ◆ Unlike subjective tinnitus, the sounds in objective tinnitus can be detected by a healthcare provider using a stethoscope or other listening devices during a physical examination.

→ **Associated Symptoms**:
  ◆ Depending on the underlying cause, objective tinnitus may be accompanied by other symptoms such as hearing loss, dizziness, or fullness in the ear.

Somatic Tinnitus

Connection with Physical Movement

Somatic tinnitus is a type of tinnitus that is influenced or modulated by physical movements or changes in the body. This form of tinnitus is often related to musculoskeletal or neurological issues and can be directly affected by actions such as head or neck movements, jaw clenching, or changes in posture.

<u>**Causes**</u>

→ **Temporomandibular Joint (TMJ) Disorders**:
- ◆ Disorders of the TMJ, which connects the jaw to the skull, can cause somatic tinnitus. Movements such as jaw clenching, chewing, or opening the mouth wide can alter the intensity or pitch of the tinnitus.

→ **Neck Problems**:
- ◆ **Cervical Spine Issues**: Conditions affecting the cervical spine, such as cervical spondylosis or neck injuries, can

lead to somatic tinnitus. Movements like turning the head or neck can change the tinnitus sounds.

◆ **Muscle Tension**: Tension in the neck and shoulder muscles can influence tinnitus, often linked to stress or poor posture.

→ **Dental Issues**:

◆ Dental problems such as misaligned teeth, bruxism (teeth grinding), or recent dental work can contribute to somatic tinnitus. Adjustments to the bite or jaw position can affect tinnitus.

→ **Neurological Disorders**:

◆ **Cranial Nerve Involvement**: Issues with cranial nerves, particularly the trigeminal or facial nerves, can cause somatic tinnitus. Movements or pressure on these nerves can modulate tinnitus sounds.

Characteristics

→ **Perceived Sounds**:
- The sounds in somatic tinnitus are similar to those in other forms of tinnitus, including ringing, buzzing, hissing, or clicking. However, these sounds are distinct in that they change in response to physical movements or manipulations.

→ **Modulation by Movement**:
- Somatic tinnitus is characterized by its sensitivity to physical movements. Actions such as moving the head, neck, or jaw; changing posture; or applying pressure to specific areas can alter the volume, pitch, or intensity of the tinnitus.

→ **Localization**:
- Somatic tinnitus can be unilateral or bilateral, depending on the underlying

cause and the affected body parts.

→ **Associated Symptoms**:
  ◆ Individuals with somatic tinnitus may also experience neck pain, jaw discomfort, headaches, or other musculoskeletal symptoms. These additional symptoms can help in diagnosing the underlying cause.

<u>Pulsatile Tinnitus</u>

Causes and Characteristics

Pulsatile tinnitus is a unique form of tinnitus characterized by a rhythmic pulsing or whooshing sound that often coincides with the person's heartbeat. Unlike other forms of tinnitus, which are typically constant and unchanging, pulsatile tinnitus has a rhythmic quality. It can be a sign of underlying vascular or blood flow-related conditions.

<u>**Causes**</u>

→ **Vascular Disorders**:
- ◆ **Atherosclerosis**: The buildup of fatty deposits in the arteries (atherosclerosis) can cause blood flow to become turbulent, leading to pulsatile tinnitus. This is often heard as a rhythmic, pulsing sound.
- ◆ **Arteriovenous Malformations (AVMs)**: Abnormal connections between arteries and veins can create turbulent blood flow, resulting in pulsatile tinnitus.
- ◆ **Carotid Artery Stenosis**: Narrowing or blockage of the carotid arteries can cause turbulent blood flow, producing a rhythmic sound in the ear.
- ◆ **Venous Hum**: Increased blood flow in the jugular vein or other large veins near the ear can cause a humming or whooshing

sound that matches the heartbeat.

→ **High Blood Pressure (Hypertension)**:
- ◆ Elevated blood pressure can increase the force of blood flow through the vessels near the ear, causing a pulsating sound.

→ **Vascular Tumors**:
- ◆ **Glomus Tumors**: These benign tumors, also known as paragangliomas, can develop in the ear or near the base of the skull and create a pulsatile tinnitus due to their blood supply and location.
- ◆ **Hemangiomas**: Benign vascular tumors that can form in the ear or surrounding areas and cause pulsatile tinnitus.

→ **Eustachian Tube Dysfunction**:
- ◆ When the eustachian tube remains open (patulous eustachian tube), it can transmit

internal sounds such as breathing and heartbeat to the ear, resulting in pulsatile tinnitus.

→ **Intracranial Hypertension**:

◆ Elevated pressure within the skull (idiopathic intracranial hypertension) can lead to pulsatile tinnitus. This condition is more common in overweight individuals, particularly women of childbearing age.

→ **Anemia**:

◆ A low red blood cell count can cause the heart to pump harder to supply enough oxygen, resulting in increased blood flow and a pulsatile sound in the ears.

Characteristics

→ **Perceived Sounds**:

◆ The hallmark of pulsatile tinnitus is a rhythmic pulsing or whooshing sound that synchronizes with the person's heartbeat. It may be described as a thumping, swooshing, or beating noise.

→ **Localization**:

◆ Pulsatile tinnitus can be unilateral (one ear) or bilateral (both ears), depending on the underlying cause. It is often more noticeable at night or in quiet environments when other sounds are absent.

→ **Detectability**:

◆ In some cases, the pulsating sound can be heard by an examiner using a stethoscope placed near the ear or over the blood vessels in the neck. This makes pulsatile tinnitus different from most other types of tinnitus, which are typically only heard by the affected individual.

→ **Associated Symptoms**:

◆ Depending on the underlying cause, pulsatile tinnitus may be accompanied by other symptoms such as headaches, dizziness, hearing loss, or a feeling of fullness in the ear. These additional symptoms can help in diagnosing the condition.

Diagnosis and Evaluation

1. Medical History and Physical Examination: A detailed medical history and thorough physical examination are crucial. The doctor will ask about the onset, duration, and nature of the tinnitus, as well as any associated symptoms and potential risk factors such as high blood pressure or recent head trauma.

2. Imaging Studies:

- **Magnetic Resonance Imaging (MRI)**: An MRI can help identify structural abnormalities, tumors, or vascular issues that may be causing pulsatile tinnitus.

- **Magnetic Resonance Angiography (MRA)** and **Computed Tomography Angiography (CTA)**: These imaging tests specifically focus on the blood vessels to detect any abnormalities or blockages.

- **Ultrasound**: Doppler ultrasound of the carotid arteries can help assess blood flow and detect any narrowing or blockages.

3. Hearing Tests: Audiometry tests can help evaluate hearing function and determine if there is any associated hearing loss.

4. Blood Tests: Blood tests may be conducted to check for conditions such as anemia or thyroid problems that could contribute to pulsatile tinnitus.

Understanding the causes and characteristics of pulsatile tinnitus is essential for accurate diagnosis and effective treatment. By identifying the underlying vascular or other medical issues, healthcare providers can develop a targeted treatment plan to alleviate the symptoms and address the root cause of pulsatile tinnitus.

CHAPTER 4:

Risk Factors and Triggers

Tinnitus affects individuals across various demographics, but certain age groups and genders are more prone to experiencing this condition. Understanding these patterns can help identify those at higher risk and tailor preventive and therapeutic strategies accordingly.

1.Age:

- **Older Adults**: Tinnitus is more prevalent in older adults, particularly those over the age of 60. Age-related hearing loss (presbycusis) is a significant contributing factor. As people age, the cumulative exposure to noise, ototoxic medications, and other health conditions increases the likelihood of developing tinnitus.
- **Middle-Aged Adults**: People in their 40s and 50s are also commonly

affected. This age group often has a combination of noise exposure from their youth and the onset of age-related hearing decline.

- **Younger Adults and Teenagers**: While less common, tinnitus can occur in younger adults and teenagers, often due to exposure to loud music, recreational noise (such as concerts and clubs), or ear infections. Increasingly, the use of personal audio devices at high volumes is becoming a significant risk factor.

2. Gender:

- **Men**: Studies indicate that men are more likely to experience tinnitus than women. This disparity may be attributed to higher rates of noise exposure among men, often due to occupational hazards and recreational activities.
- **Women**: While less prevalent, tinnitus in women is not uncommon

and can be linked to factors such as hormonal changes (e.g., menopause), stress, and anxiety, which can exacerbate tinnitus symptoms.

3. Environmental Factors

Noise Exposure

One of the most significant environmental risk factors for tinnitus is noise exposure. Both acute and chronic exposure to loud sounds can damage the delicate hair cells in the inner ear, leading to hearing loss and tinnitus.

→ **Loud Music**:
  - ◆ Exposure to loud music at concerts, clubs, or through personal audio devices can cause temporary or permanent hearing damage. High decibel levels, especially over extended periods, can lead to tinnitus.

→ **Workplace Noise**:

◆ Certain occupations expose individuals to continuous loud noise, such as construction workers, factory employees, musicians, and military personnel. Long-term exposure without adequate hearing protection can result in tinnitus and hearing loss.

→ **Recreational Noise**:

◆ Activities such as hunting, shooting, and using power tools or loud machinery can also contribute to noise-induced tinnitus. Proper use of ear protection is essential to mitigate this risk.

→ **Sudden Loud Noises**:

◆ Exposure to sudden loud noises, such as explosions or gunfire, can cause immediate hearing damage and acute tinnitus. This type of exposure is common in military settings and among individuals involved in explosive demolition work.

4. Occupational Hazards

Occupational hazards play a significant role in the development of tinnitus. Certain work environments expose individuals to high noise levels, chemicals, and other factors that can increase the risk of tinnitus.

→ **High-Noise Environments**:
   ◆ Occupations in construction, manufacturing, agriculture, and the military often involve exposure to loud machinery, engines, and equipment. Prolonged exposure without proper hearing protection can lead to chronic tinnitus.

→ **Musicians and Entertainment Industry Workers**:
   ◆ Musicians, DJs, and sound engineers are frequently exposed to high decibel levels during

performances and recordings. Continuous exposure to loud music without adequate hearing protection increases the risk of tinnitus.

→ **Aviation Industry**:

◆ Pilots, flight attendants, and ground crew in the aviation industry are exposed to high levels of noise from aircraft engines and equipment. Hearing protection is crucial in these environments to prevent tinnitus and hearing loss.

→ **Military Personnel**:

◆ Military service members are at significant risk of tinnitus due to exposure to gunfire, explosions, and loud machinery. Tinnitus is one of the most common service-related disabilities among veterans.

→ **Factory and Industrial Workers**:

◆ Workers in factories and industrial settings may be exposed to continuous noise from heavy machinery, press machines, and other equipment. Hearing conservation programs and the use of protective devices are vital in these settings.

5. Lifestyle Factors

Diet and Exercise

Diet and **exercise** play crucial roles in overall health and can significantly impact the severity and perception of tinnitus.

→ **Diet**:

◆ **Nutritional Balance**: A balanced diet rich in vitamins and minerals supports overall ear health. Foods high in antioxidants, such as fruits and vegetables, can help reduce inflammation and oxidative stress, which may influence tinnitus.

◆ **Specific Nutrients**: Certain nutrients, like magnesium, zinc, and vitamin B12, are linked to hearing health. Deficiencies in these nutrients may exacerbate tinnitus symptoms.

◆ **Salt Intake**: High sodium levels can lead to increased blood pressure, potentially worsening tinnitus. Reducing salt intake may help alleviate symptoms for some individuals.

◆ **Caffeine and Alcohol**: These substances can impact blood flow and may worsen tinnitus for some people. Monitoring intake and reducing consumption may provide relief.

◆ **Hydration**: Staying well-hydrated is essential for overall health. Dehydration can lead to reduced blood flow, potentially affecting tinnitus symptoms.

→ **Exercise**:

◆ **Physical Activity**: Regular exercise improves circulation and helps reduce stress, which can positively affect tinnitus. Activities such as walking, swimming, or cycling can be beneficial.

◆ **Stress Reduction**: Exercise is an effective way to manage stress and anxiety, both of which can worsen tinnitus symptoms. Engaging in physical activity releases endorphins, improving mood and overall well-being.

◆ **Balance and Coordination**: Certain exercises, like yoga or tai chi, can improve balance and reduce feelings of dizziness associated with tinnitus.

Stress and Anxiety

Stress and **anxiety** are significant lifestyle factors that can exacerbate tinnitus symptoms. Understanding their impact is crucial for effective management.

→ **Psychological Impact**:
- ◆ Tinnitus can create a cycle of stress and anxiety. The perception of sound can lead to frustration, which can, in turn, increase stress levels and make the tinnitus feel louder or more intrusive.

→ **Stress Response**:
- ◆ When under stress, the body releases hormones such as cortisol, which can affect blood flow and alter the perception of sound. Chronic stress can heighten sensitivity to tinnitus.

→ **Coping Strategies**:
- ◆ **Mindfulness and Relaxation Techniques**: Practices such as meditation, deep breathing, and progressive muscle relaxation

can help reduce stress and improve the ability to cope with tinnitus.

◆ **Therapy and Counseling**: Cognitive-behavioral therapy (CBT) and other therapeutic approaches can assist individuals in developing coping strategies for managing stress and anxiety related to tinnitus.

→ **Sleep Quality**:

◆ Stress and anxiety can lead to sleep disturbances, which can exacerbate tinnitus symptoms. Establishing a consistent sleep routine and creating a calming sleep environment can improve both sleep quality and tinnitus perception.

By addressing lifestyle factors such as diet, exercise, stress, and anxiety, individuals can take proactive steps to manage their tinnitus more effectively. Integrating healthy habits into daily life can contribute to overall well-being and potentially reduce the impact of tinnitus on quality of life.

CHAPTER 5:

Medical and Surgical Treatments

Types of Drugs Used

Medications can play a significant role in managing tinnitus, although no specific drug is universally effective. Various types of drugs are used to address underlying conditions, reduce symptoms, or improve overall quality of life for individuals with tinnitus.

- ❖ **<u>Antidepressants</u>:**
    - ➤ **Examples**: Amitriptyline, Nortriptyline, Sertraline.
    - ➤ **Purpose**: Often prescribed to help manage anxiety and depression, which can accompany tinnitus. They may also help alleviate tinnitus symptoms for some individuals.

- ❖ **<u>Anti-anxiety Medications</u>**:
  - ➤ **Examples**: Diazepam, Clonazepam.
  - ➤ **Purpose**: These can reduce anxiety levels and may provide temporary relief from tinnitus symptoms, especially in individuals with high stress.
- ❖ **<u>Anticonvulsants</u>**:
  - ➤ **Examples**: Gabapentin, Pregabalin.
  - ➤ **Purpose**: Sometimes used to help manage nerve-related pain and may have a positive effect on tinnitus, particularly in patients with neuropathic pain.
- ❖ **<u>Corticosteroids</u>**:
  - ➤ **Examples**: Prednisone.
  - ➤ **Purpose**: These may be prescribed for sudden onset tinnitus related to inner ear inflammation or injury. Their effectiveness can vary depending on the underlying cause.

- ❖ <u>**Zinc Supplements**</u>:
  - ➢ **Purpose**: Some studies suggest that zinc may help reduce tinnitus symptoms in individuals with a deficiency, although evidence is mixed.
- ❖ <u>**Baclofen**</u>:
  - ➢ **Purpose**: Muscle relaxants like baclofen may help in cases where muscle tension contributes to tinnitus.
- ❖ <u>**Sound-Generating Devices**</u>:
  - ➢ **Purpose**: While not medications per se, devices that generate white noise or other sounds can help mask tinnitus, making it less noticeable.

Effectiveness and Side Effects

The effectiveness of medications for tinnitus can vary significantly among individuals, and it's essential to consider potential side effects.

→ **Effectiveness**:

- ◆ **Variable Results**: Some patients report significant relief from tinnitus symptoms with certain medications, while others may experience little to no change. It often requires trial and error to find an effective treatment.
- ◆ **Adjunctive Therapy**: Medications are typically used as part of a broader treatment strategy, including sound therapy and counseling, rather than as standalone solutions.

→ **Side Effects**:

- ◆ **Antidepressants**: Common side effects can include weight gain, dry mouth, dizziness, and fatigue. Some individuals may also experience an increase in suicidal thoughts, particularly in younger patients.

- ◆ **Anti-anxiety Medications**: Side effects may include drowsiness, dizziness, dependence, and withdrawal symptoms when discontinuing use.
- ◆ **Anticonvulsants**: Side effects can include dizziness, drowsiness, and coordination problems. Long-term use may require monitoring for additional side effects.
- ◆ **Corticosteroids**: Potential side effects include increased blood pressure, weight gain, mood changes, and increased risk of infection with long-term use.
- ◆ **Zinc Supplements**: High doses can lead to nausea, vomiting, and other gastrointestinal issues.

While medications can provide relief for some individuals with tinnitus, they are not a solution that works for everyone. Working closely with a healthcare provider is essential to tailor treatment plans to each individual's needs, monitor effectiveness, and manage any side effects. Combining medications with other therapeutic approaches, such as cognitive-behavioral therapy and sound therapy, often yields the best results for managing tinnitus.

Sound Therapy

1. Masking Devices

Masking devices are tools designed to help individuals cope with tinnitus by producing external sounds to cover or mask the internal sounds of tinnitus.

Functionality:

These devices emit white noise or other soothing sounds to help distract the brain from the tinnitus. This can make the perception of tinnitus less intrusive, especially in quiet environments.

Types of Masking Devices:

- **Tabletop Devices**: Standalone machines that generate sound, often used during sleep or in quiet spaces.

- **Wearable Devices**: Similar to hearing aids, these fit in or over the ear and provide a constant sound to mask tinnitus throughout the day.

- **Smartphone Apps**: Many apps offer sound therapy options, allowing users to play various sounds or white noise directly from their phones.

Effectiveness:

Many users report a significant reduction in the perception of tinnitus when using masking devices, particularly during quiet times or when trying to sleep.

Limitations:

While masking devices can be effective, they do not eliminate tinnitus. Some individuals may need additional therapy or support to address underlying causes or emotional impacts.

2. Hearing Aids

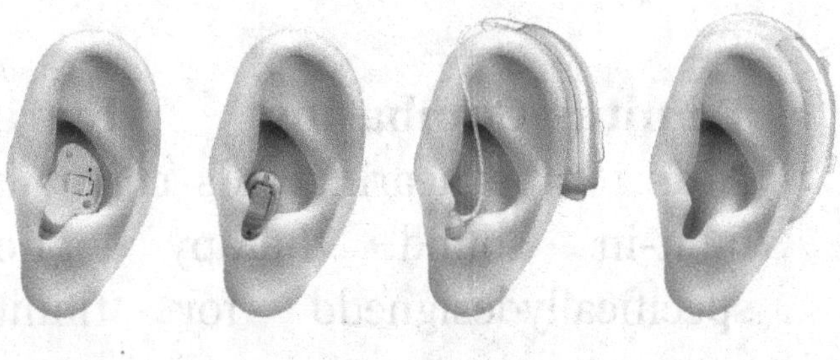

Hearing aids can be beneficial for individuals with tinnitus, especially those who also experience hearing loss.

Dual Functionality: Hearing aids amplify external sounds, which can help mask tinnitus sounds and make them less noticeable. This is particularly effective in noisy environments.

Types of Hearing Aids:

- **Traditional Hearing Aids**: Designed primarily for hearing loss, these devices can also assist with tinnitus by providing background noise.

- **Tinnitus-Combating Hearing Aids**: Some hearing aids come with built-in sound therapy options specificallydesignedd for tinnitus management.

Effectiveness:

Many users find that hearing aids significantly reduce the perception of tinnitus, improve communication, and enhance overall quality of life.

Limitations:

Hearing aids may not work for everyone, particularly those with normal hearing who experience tinnitus. Additionally, they can be costly and may require time to adjust to.

Surgical Options

When Surgery is Considered

Surgery is not a common treatment for tinnitus but may be considered in specific cases, particularly when there is an identifiable underlying condition that can be corrected surgically.

❖ **Indications for Surgery**:
> **Objective Tinnitus**: If tinnitus is caused by a structural issue, such as a vascular malformation or a tumor, surgery may be an appropriate option.

> **Severe Cases**: In cases where tinnitus significantly affects quality of life and other treatments have failed, surgical intervention may be considered.

Types of Surgeries and Outcomes

❖ **Vascular Surgery**:

> ➢ **Arteriovenous Malformation (AVM) Removal**: Surgical intervention to remove an AVM can alleviate pulsatile tinnitus caused by abnormal blood flow.

> ➢ **Carotid Artery Surgery**: In cases of carotid artery stenosis, surgical correction can reduce tinnitus related to turbulent blood flow.

❖ **Tumor Removal**:

> ➢ **Glomus Tumor Surgery**: Removing benign tumors in the ear can resolve tinnitus caused by these growths. Outcomes are

generally positive, with many patients experiencing significant relief post-surgery.

- ❖ **Middle Ear Surgery**:
  - ➢ **Stapedectomy**: This procedure can improve hearing and may relieve tinnitus in certain cases by addressing middle ear dysfunction.
- ❖ **Cochlear Implants**:
  - ➢ For individuals with profound hearing loss and tinnitus, cochlear implants can provide access to sound, which may help mask tinnitus and improve overall auditory function.

Outcomes and Considerations

- → **Effectiveness**:
  - ◆ Surgical outcomes vary widely depending on the underlying condition, with some patients experiencing complete

resolution of tinnitus and others seeing little to no change.

→ **Risks and Complications**:

◆ As with any surgery, there are inherent risks, including infection, bleeding, and potential worsening of tinnitus. Patients must weigh the potential benefits against these risks.

→ **Postoperative Care**:

◆ Ongoing follow-up and care are essential after surgery to monitor recovery and address any complications or persistent symptoms.

In summary, while sound therapy options like masking devices and hearing aids can provide relief for many individuals with tinnitus, surgical options may be appropriate for specific underlying conditions. A comprehensive evaluation by a healthcare professional is crucial in determining the most suitable treatment approach.

CHAPTER 6:

Alternative and Complementary Therapies

Herbal Remedies

Herbal remedies have gained popularity among individuals seeking alternative treatments for tinnitus. While some supplements may show promise, it's essential to approach these therapies with caution and consult a healthcare provider before starting any new regimen.

Common Supplements and Their Efficacy

1. **<u>Ginkgo Biloba</u>:**

Description: An herbal extract derived from the leaves of the Ginkgo tree, traditionally used for cognitive enhancement and circulatory issues.

Efficacy: Some studies suggest that Ginkgo biloba may help alleviate tinnitus symptoms by improving blood flow to the inner ear. However, results are mixed, and more research is needed to confirm its effectiveness.

2. <u>Zinc</u>:

Description: An essential mineral that plays a crucial role in immune function and cellular metabolism.

Efficacy: Zinc supplementation has been studied for its potential benefits in tinnitus, particularly in individuals with zinc deficiency. Some studies indicate that it may reduce symptoms, but more robust research is required to establish conclusive results.

3. <u>Magnesium</u>:

Description: A vital mineral involved in many biochemical reactions in the body, including nerve function and muscle contraction.

Efficacy: Magnesium may help protect the inner ear from damage caused by excessive noise exposure and is thought to reduce the severity of tinnitus in some individuals. Evidence is still emerging, highlighting the need for further studies.

4. <u>Vitamin B12</u>:

Description: A water-soluble vitamin essential for nerve function and the production of red blood cells.

Efficacy: Some research suggests a link between vitamin B12 deficiency and tinnitus. Supplementation may benefit those with low levels, but further studies are necessary to confirm this connection.

5. <u>Niacin (Vitamin B3)</u>:

Description: Another B vitamin involved in energy metabolism and circulation.

Efficacy: Niacin is believed to improve blood flow, which could theoretically help with tinnitus. However, evidence is limited, and high doses can cause side effects such as flushing and gastrointestinal upset.

6. <u>Folic Acid</u>:

Description: A B vitamin important for cell division and the synthesis of DNA.

Efficacy: Some studies suggest that folic acid may help reduce the risk of tinnitus, particularly in older adults. More research is needed to establish its role in treatment.

7. <u>Herbal Blends</u>:

Description: Various herbal combinations marketed for tinnitus relief, often containing ingredients like Ginkgo biloba, zinc, and B vitamins.

Efficacy: The effectiveness of these blends varies, and while some users report relief, scientific evidence supporting their use is often lacking.

Considerations for Using Herbal Remedies

1.Consultation with Healthcare Providers:It's crucial to consult a healthcare professional before starting any herbal supplements, especially if you are taking other medications or have underlying health conditions.

2. Quality and Regulation: Herbal supplements are not as tightly regulated as prescription medications, leading to variability in quality and potency. It's essential to choose products from reputable manufacturers to ensure safety and efficacy.

3. Potential Side Effects: Herbal remedies can cause side effects and interact with other medications. Awareness of these potential issues is vital to avoid adverse reactions.

4. Individual Variability: The effectiveness of herbal remedies can vary widely among individuals. What works for one person may not work for another, and it may take time to determine the right approach.

While some herbal remedies show promise for managing tinnitus symptoms, more research is needed to establish their effectiveness conclusively. Individuals considering these therapies should do so with caution, under the guidance of a healthcare provider, and as part of a comprehensive treatment strategy that includes traditional medical approaches when necessary.

Acupuncture

How It Works

Acupuncture is an ancient Chinese healing practice that involves inserting thin needles into specific points on the body to stimulate energy flow and promote healing.

→ **Principles of Acupuncture:**

◆ Based on Traditional Chinese Medicine (TCM), acupuncture aims to balance the body's energy, or "Qi" (pronounced "chee"), which is believed to flow through meridians (energy pathways).
◆ Practitioners target specific acupuncture points to address various health issues, including pain, stress, and tinnitus.

→ **Procedure**:
◆ A licensed acupuncturist conducts an assessment, identifying relevant points based on the individual's symptoms.
◆ Needles are inserted into specific points, often causing minimal discomfort. The duration and number of sessions vary depending on the treatment plan.

Evidence and Effectiveness

* ❖ **Research Findings**:
  * ➢ Some studies suggest that acupuncture may provide relief for tinnitus, particularly in cases related to stress or anxiety. However, evidence remains mixed, and more rigorous research is needed.
  * ➢ A systematic review of studies found that acupuncture might be more effective than placebo treatments but less so compared to conventional therapies.
* ❖ **Limitations**:
  * ➢ Results can vary widely among individuals, and not all patients experience relief from tinnitus through acupuncture.
  * ➢ The quality of studies varies, and some may suffer from methodological limitations, making it challenging to draw definitive conclusions.

Mind-Body Techniques

Mind-body techniques focus on the connection between mental and physical health and can play a valuable role in managing tinnitus symptoms.

Meditation

→ **How It Works**:

- ◆ Meditation involves training the mind to focus and redirect thoughts, often promoting relaxation and reducing stress.
- ◆ Techniques may include mindfulness meditation, which encourages awareness of thoughts and sensations without judgment.

→ **Benefits for Tinnitus**:

- ◆ Research indicates that meditation can help reduce stress and anxiety levels, which can contribute to the perception of tinnitus.

◆ Many individuals report feeling calmer and more in control of their tinnitus symptoms through regular meditation practice.

Yoga and Relaxation Techniques

→ **Yoga**:

◆ Combines physical postures, breathing exercises, and meditation to promote relaxation and overall well-being.

◆ Regular practice can improve flexibility, reduce stress, and enhance mental clarity.

→ **Benefits for Tinnitus**:

◆ Yoga can help alleviate the physical tension and stress that may worsen tinnitus symptoms. Many practitioners report improvements in their overall quality of life and reduced awareness of tinnitus.

→ **Relaxation Techniques**:

◆ Techniques such as progressive muscle relaxation, deep breathing exercises, and guided imagery can help manage stress and promote relaxation.

◆ These practices can provide immediate relief from anxiety related to tinnitus and help create a more positive mental state.

Alternative therapies like acupuncture and mind-body techniques can be valuable components of a comprehensive tinnitus management plan. While evidence supporting their effectiveness varies, many individuals find these approaches helpful in reducing stress and improving overall well-being. As always, it's essential to consult healthcare professionals before starting any new treatment regimen to ensure safety and appropriateness.

CHAPTER 7:

Coping Strategies and Lifestyle Adjustments

Managing Stress and Anxiety

Stress and anxiety can significantly amplify the perception of tinnitus, making effective management crucial for improving quality of life. Here are some techniques and practices to help manage these feelings:

Techniques and Practices

→ **Mindfulness Meditation:**
- ◆ **Description**: Mindfulness involves being present in the moment and observing thoughts without judgment.
- ◆ **Practice**: Set aside a few minutes each day to focus on your breath or the sounds around you. This practice can help reduce anxiety and increase

awareness of tinnitus, allowing for greater acceptance.

→ **Deep Breathing Exercises**:

  ◆ **Description**: Deep breathing helps calm the nervous system and reduce physical tension.

  ◆ **Practice**: Try the 4-7-8 technique: inhale for 4 seconds, hold for 7 seconds, and exhale for 8 seconds. Repeat several times to promote relaxation.

→ **Progressive Muscle Relaxation (PMR)**:

  ◆ **Description**: PMR involves systematically tensing and then relaxing different muscle groups to alleviate tension.

  ◆ **Practice**: Start from your toes and work your way up to your head, tensing each muscle group for a few seconds before relaxing. This can help relieve physical stress related to tinnitus.

→ **Cognitive Behavioral Therapy (CBT)**:
- ◆ **Description**: CBT is a structured form of therapy that helps individuals identify and change negative thought patterns related to tinnitus.
- ◆ **Practice**: Working with a trained therapist can provide tools to cope with tinnitus and reduce its emotional impact.

→ **Exercise**:
- ◆ **Description**: Regular physical activity can lower stress and anxiety levels, improve mood, and enhance overall well-being.
- ◆ **Practice**: Aim for at least 30 minutes of moderate exercise most days of the week. Activities like walking, swimming, or yoga can be particularly beneficial.

→ **Journaling**:
- ◆ **Description**: Writing about thoughts and feelings can

provide an outlet for stress and help process emotions related to tinnitus.

◆ **Practice**: Set aside time each day to jot down your experiences, worries, and coping strategies. This can help clarify thoughts and reduce anxiety.

→ **Support Groups**:

◆ **Description**: Connecting with others who experience tinnitus can provide emotional support and practical advice.

◆ **Practice**: Join a local or online support group to share experiences, learn from others, and gain encouragement.

→ **Healthy Lifestyle Choices**:

◆ **Description**: Maintaining a balanced diet, getting enough sleep, and limiting alcohol and caffeine can positively impact stress levels.

◆ **Practice**: Focus on whole foods, regular sleep patterns, and hydration to support overall health and mitigate tinnitus symptoms.

→ **Sound Therapy**:

◆ **Description**: Using background noise or soothing sounds can help mask tinnitus and promote relaxation.

◆ **Practice**: Consider using white noise machines, apps, or gentle music to create a calming environment that reduces awareness of tinnitus.

→ **Mindful Movement**:

◆ **Description**: Practices like yoga and tai chi combine movement with mindfulness, promoting relaxation and reducing stress.

◆ **Practice**: make these activities part of your routine to foster both physical and mental well-being.

Managing stress and anxiety is vital for coping with tinnitus. By integrating these techniques and practices into their daily lives, individuals can create a more balanced approach to managing their condition. Emphasizing self-care and emotional well-being can lead to improved quality of life and a better ability to cope with the challenges of tinnitus.

Diet and Nutrition

Diet and nutrition play an essential role in managing tinnitus symptoms. Certain foods can help alleviate symptoms, while others may exacerbate them. Here's a closer look at foods that may help or harm.

Foods That May Help

- ❖ **Fruits and Vegetables**:
    - ➢ **Benefits**: Rich in antioxidants, vitamins, and minerals, these

foods can support overall health and reduce inflammation.

> **Examples**: Berries, leafy greens, and citrus fruits are particularly beneficial.

❖ **Whole Grains**:

> **Benefits**: Whole grains provide steady energy and are linked to improved heart health, which may help with circulation and ear health.

> **Examples**: Brown rice, quinoa, oats, and whole-grain bread.

❖ **Lean Proteins**:

> **Benefits**: Protein supports tissue repair and overall health. Lean sources can help maintain a balanced diet without excessive fat.

> **Examples**: Chicken, turkey, fish, beans, and legumes.

❖ **Healthy Fats**:

> **Benefits**: Omega-3 fatty acids have anti-inflammatory

properties that may support ear health.

> **Examples**: Fatty fish (salmon, mackerel), walnuts, and flaxseeds.

❖ **Nuts and Seeds**:

> **Benefits**: These are good sources of vitamins and minerals, including zinc and magnesium, which may help with tinnitus symptoms.

> **Examples**: Almonds, sunflower seeds, and pumpkin seeds.

❖ **Herbs and Spices**:

> **Benefits**: Certain herbs and spices can have anti-inflammatory effects and promote circulation.

> **Examples**: Garlic, ginger, and turmeric.

❖ **Hydration**:

> **Benefits**: Staying hydrated is crucial for overall health, including ear function.

> ➤ **Recommendation**: Aim for adequate water intake throughout the day.

Foods That May Harm

- ❖ **Caffeine**:
    - ➤ **Effects**: Caffeine can increase anxiety and may exacerbate tinnitus symptoms for some individuals.
    - ➤ **Sources**: Coffee, tea, energy drinks, and certain sodas.
- ❖ **Alcohol**:
    - ➤ **Effects**: Alcohol can affect blood flow and may worsen tinnitus symptoms.
    - ➤ **Recommendation**: Limit or avoid alcoholic beverages, particularly if symptoms increase after consumption.
- ❖ **Salt**:
    - ➤ **Effects**: High sodium intake can lead to fluid retention, potentially increasing pressure

in the inner ear and exacerbating tinnitus.

> **Sources**: Processed foods, canned soups, and salty snacks.

❖ **Sugary Foods**:

> **Effects**: High sugar intake may lead to increased inflammation and negative health impacts that could affect tinnitus.

> **Sources**: Sweets, sugary drinks, and processed snacks.

❖ **Processed Foods**:

> **Effects**: These often contain unhealthy fats, high sodium, and additives that may negatively affect overall health and tinnitus symptoms.

> **Sources**: Fast food, packaged snacks, and ready-to-eat meals.

❖ **Aspartame**:

> **Effects**: Some individuals report worsening tinnitus symptoms after consuming

aspartame, an artificial sweetener.
> **Sources**: Diet sodas, sugar-free products, and certain candies.

Diet and nutrition can significantly impact tinnitus management. By incorporating beneficial foods and avoiding harmful ones, individuals can support their overall health and potentially reduce tinnitus symptoms. A balanced diet, rich in whole foods and low in processed ingredients, is key to promoting well-being and managing the challenges associated with tinnitus.

Sleep Management

Improving Sleep Quality with Tinnitus

Getting quality sleep is crucial for overall health and well-being, especially for those dealing with tinnitus. Here are strategies to improve sleep quality despite the presence of tinnitus:

1. Establish a Consistent Sleep Routine:

Tip: Go to bed and wake up at the same time each day to regulate your body's internal clock.

Benefit: A consistent schedule can improve sleep quality and reduce insomnia.

2. Create a Comfortable Sleep Environment:

Tip: Ensure your bedroom is dark, quiet, and cool. Consider using blackout curtains and earplugs or white noise machines to block out disturbances.

Benefit: A conducive environment can help mask tinnitus sounds and promote relaxation.

3. Sound Therapy:

Tip: Use soft background sounds, such as white noise or nature sounds, to help mask tinnitus while sleeping.

Benefit: Sound therapy can make tinnitus less noticeable and aid in falling asleep.

4. Limit Stimulants:

Tip: Avoid caffeine and nicotine, especially in the hours leading up to bedtime.

Benefit: Reducing stimulants can improve your ability to fall asleep and stay asleep.

5. Relaxation Techniques:

Tip: Engage in calming activities before bed, such as reading, gentle stretching, or deep breathing exercises.

Benefit: Relaxation techniques can help reduce anxiety and prepare your mind for sleep.

6. Avoid Heavy Meals Before Bed:

Tip: Refrain from eating large meals or spicy foods close to bedtime.

Benefit: A light snack may be fine, but heavy meals can lead to discomfort and disrupt sleep.

7. Limit Screen Time:

Tip: Reduce exposure to screens (phones, tablets, TVs) at least an hour before bed.

Benefit: The blue light emitted by screens can interfere with melatonin production and disrupt sleep patterns.

Social and Emotional Support

Importance of Support Networks

Having a strong support network is essential for individuals coping with tinnitus. Emotional and social support can provide reassurance and help manage the condition more effectively.

1.Emotional Resilience:

Tip: Sharing experiences and challenges with others can foster emotional resilience.

Benefit: Knowing you're not alone can alleviate feelings of isolation and anxiety.

2. Practical Advice:

Tip: Support networks can offer practical tips and coping strategies based on personal experiences.

Benefit: Learning from others can provide new insights into managing tinnitus.

3. Encouragement:

Tip: Supportive friends and family can offer encouragement during difficult times.

Benefit: Positive reinforcement can boost motivation and help individuals maintain a proactive approach to managing tinnitus.

Support Groups and Counseling

→ **Support Groups**:
- ◆ **Description**: Joining a support group can connect individuals

with others who understand their experiences with tinnitus.

◆ **Benefits**:

- Provides a safe space to share feelings and experiences.
- Offers opportunities to learn about different coping strategies and treatments.

→ **Counseling**:

◆ **Description**: Professional counseling can provide structured support and coping strategies tailored to individual needs.

◆ **Benefits**:

- Therapists can help address emotional challenges related to tinnitus, such as anxiety and depression.
- Counseling can teach techniques like Cognitive

Behavioral Therapy (CBT) to manage negative thought patterns.

Effective sleep management and strong social support are vital components of coping with tinnitus. By implementing strategies to improve sleep quality and seeking emotional support from networks or professional counseling, individuals can enhance their overall well-being and resilience in the face of tinnitus challenges.

CHAPTER 8:

Technological Advances and Future Directions

Innovative Treatments

As our understanding of tinnitus evolves, so do the technological advancements aimed at treating this condition. Here are two significant innovations making waves in tinnitus management.

<u>Neuromodulation</u>

What is Neuromodulation?

Neuromodulation involves using electrical or magnetic stimulation to alter nerve activity in the brain, aiming to change how the brain perceives tinnitus.

How It Works:

Neuromodulation techniques, such as transcranial magnetic stimulation (TMS) and transcranial direct current stimulation (tDCS), target specific brain regions involved in auditory processing and tinnitus perception.

Benefits:

- Early research suggests that neuromodulation can lead to a reduction in tinnitus severity and improved quality of life for some patients.
- It may also promote neuroplasticity, enabling the brain to adapt and potentially lessen tinnitus symptoms over time.

Current Research and Future Directions:

Ongoing studies are exploring optimal stimulation parameters, long-term effectiveness, and the best patient profiles for these treatments.

As technology advances, personalized neuromodulation protocols may become more widely available, offering tailored solutions for tinnitus sufferers.

Cochlear Implants

What are Cochlear Implants?

Cochlear implants are electronic devices that bypass damaged portions of the ear and directly stimulate the auditory nerve, providing a sense of sound to individuals with severe hearing loss or deafness.

How They Help with Tinnitus:

For individuals with hearing loss, cochlear implants can reduce tinnitus symptoms by restoring some level of auditory input, which may help mask the perception of tinnitus.

Studies show that many cochlear implant users report a reduction in tinnitus severity post-implantation.

Benefits:

Cochlear implants can improve overall hearing capabilities, which can contribute to better communication and social engagement.

They offer a potential dual benefit for those who experience both hearing loss and tinnitus.

Current Research and Future Directions:

Research is ongoing to optimize cochlear implant technology and develop improved devices that better address tinnitus symptoms.

Innovations such as sound-processing strategies specifically designed for tinnitus relief are being explored, which could enhance the effectiveness of cochlear implants for tinnitus patients.

Innovative treatments such as **neuromodulation** and **<u>cochlear implants</u>** represent exciting advancements in tinnitus management. As research progresses, these technologies may offer new hope for individuals seeking relief from tinnitus symptoms, paving the way for more personalized and effective treatment options in the future.

Research and Development

As the understanding of tinnitus continues to grow, ongoing research aims to uncover new treatments and improve existing therapies. Here's a look at current studies and promising future therapies.

Current Studies and Findings

1. Neuromodulation Research:

Recent studies have focused on the efficacy of various neuromodulation techniques, such as transcranial magnetic stimulation (TMS) and transcranial direct current stimulation (tDCS). Findings indicate that these methods can lead to significant reductions in tinnitus loudness and annoyance in some patients.

2. Sound Therapy Investigations:

Research into sound therapy, including the use of white noise, music, and tailored soundscapes, has shown positive results. Studies suggest that consistent sound therapy can help desensitize the brain to tinnitus and improve patients' quality of life.

3. Cochlear Implant Studies:

Ongoing research evaluates the effectiveness of cochlear implants not only for hearing loss but also for their impact on tinnitus. Findings indicate that many users report reduced tinnitus symptoms after implantation, reinforcing the dual benefits of these devices.

4. Pharmacological Trials:

Various clinical trials are exploring medications that may help alleviate tinnitus symptoms, including antidepressants, anti-anxiety medications, and supplements. Preliminary findings suggest mixed results, emphasizing the need for further research.

5. Genetic Studies:

Emerging studies are investigating the genetic factors that may predispose individuals to tinnitus, which could lead to targeted therapies in the future. Understanding the genetic basis could help identify those at higher risk and develop preventive strategies.

Promising Future Therapies

- ❖ **Combination Therapies**:
  - ➢ Researchers are exploring combination therapies that integrate sound therapy, neuromodulation, and cognitive behavioral therapy (CBT) to create a more comprehensive

approach to tinnitus management. This holistic approach may yield better results for patients.

❖ **Personalized Medicine**:

> ➤ Advances in personalized medicine may lead to tailored treatments based on individual patient profiles, including their specific tinnitus characteristics, underlying conditions, and responses to prior therapies. Custom solutions could enhance treatment efficacy.

❖ **Biofeedback and Virtual Reality**:

> ➤ Innovative techniques like biofeedback and virtual reality are being studied for their potential to help patients manage tinnitus symptoms. These technologies aim to enhance relaxation and provide immersive experiences that distract from tinnitus.

❖ **New Devices and Apps**:
  ➤ The development of wearable devices and mobile applications designed to deliver sound therapy and track tinnitus symptoms is underway. These tools aim to provide accessible and user-friendly solutions for managing tinnitus.
❖ **Research into Neuroplasticity**:
  ➤ Future therapies may focus on promoting neuroplasticity—the brain's ability to adapt and change—through targeted exercises and therapies. This approach could help retrain the brain's response to tinnitus over time.

The landscape of tinnitus research and development is dynamic, with numerous studies exploring innovative treatments and potential breakthroughs. As ongoing research continues to yield promising findings, the future holds the possibility of more effective and personalized therapies for those affected by tinnitus, offering hope for improved quality of life and symptom management.

CHAPTER 9:

Living with Tinnitus

Personal Stories

Hearing from others who share similar experiences can be invaluable for those living with tinnitus. Personal stories can provide insight, hope, and practical coping strategies. Here are several case studies and testimonials that illustrate diverse experiences with tinnitus.

Case Studies

1. **Sarah's Journey: Finding Acceptance**

Sarah, a 34-year-old teacher, developed tinnitus after a concert exposure to loud music.

Initially overwhelmed, she struggled with anxiety and sleepless nights. After seeking help, Sarah learned about sound therapy and began using a white noise machine at night.

Over time, Sarah found that while the tinnitus was still present, she could manage her anxiety and improve her sleep quality, leading to a more positive outlook on life.

2. Mark's Path: From Isolation to Community

Mark, a 50-year-old engineer, experienced sudden onset tinnitus following a bout of ear infections.

Feeling isolated, he searched for support and discovered a local tinnitus support group. Engaging with others helped him feel less alone and provided practical coping strategies.

Mark reports that connecting with others has significantly reduced his feelings of isolation, and he now actively participates in group discussions.

3. **Emily's Approach: Integrating Mindfulness**

Emily, a 28-year-old graphic designer, developed tinnitus during a stressful period in her life.

Seeking relief, she turned to mindfulness meditation and cognitive behavioral therapy (CBT). These techniques allowed her to shift her focus away from the tinnitus.

Emily now practices mindfulness daily, and while the tinnitus remains, she has learned to manage her reactions and reduce its emotional impact.

Testimonials

1. **John's Experience with Technology**:

"After trying various treatments for my tinnitus, I finally found relief with sound therapy. Using a hearing aid with built-in sound masking features has changed my life. I can finally enjoy conversations without the constant ringing in my ears."

2. **Lisa's Journey to Understanding**:

"Living with tinnitus has been a rollercoaster. Initially, I felt hopeless, but learning more about the condition and connecting with others in a support group has empowered me. I now have tools to cope and a community that understands what I'm going through."

3. **David's Exploration of Alternatives**:

"I was skeptical about acupuncture, but after a few sessions, I noticed a significant reduction in my tinnitus symptoms. It might not work for everyone, but it has made a positive difference in my life."

Daily Life Tips

Practical Advice for Day-to-Day Management

Managing tinnitus on a daily basis can be challenging, but with practical strategies, individuals can improve their quality of life. Below are some effective tips:

1.Establish a Routine: Create a daily schedule that includes regular activities, work hours, and relaxation time. A consistent routine can help reduce anxiety and provide a sense of control.

2. Use Sound Therapy: Incorporate background noise or soothing sounds into your environment. Whether through a white noise machine, apps, or nature sounds, these can help mask tinnitus and promote relaxation.

3. Practice Stress Reduction Techniques: Engage in daily practices like deep breathing, meditation, or yoga to manage stress. Reducing stress can lead to decreased tinnitus perception and improved emotional well-being.

4. Limit Exposure to Loud Environments: Protect your ears by avoiding loud places or using earplugs when necessary. Reducing noise exposure can prevent worsening symptoms.

5. Stay Active: Regular physical activity can enhance mood and reduce stress. Aim for at least 30 minutes of exercise most days, such as walking, cycling, or swimming.

5. Connect with Others: Reach out to friends, family, or support groups. Sharing your experiences and feelings can provide emotional relief and practical advice.

6. Educate Yourself: Learn as much as possible about tinnitus. Understanding the condition can help you feel more empowered and reduce fear of the unknown.

7. Maintain a Healthy Lifestyle: Focus on a balanced diet, stay hydrated, and prioritize sleep. Healthy habits can positively impact overall well-being and may reduce tinnitus symptoms.

Balancing Work, Social Life, and Personal Well-being

Living with tinnitus requires careful attention to balance various aspects of life. Here are strategies to maintain quality of life while managing tinnitus:

1. Workplace Accommodations: Communicate with your employer about your needs. Consider flexible work arrangements or modifications to your workspace, such as noise-canceling headphones, to help you focus and reduce distractions.

2. Set Realistic Goals: Establish achievable goals for work and personal life. Break tasks into smaller steps to prevent feeling overwhelmed and to maintain motivation.

3. Social Engagement: Prioritize social interactions that uplift you. Choose quieter settings for socializing, and don't hesitate to discuss your condition with close friends who can offer understanding and support.

4. Time for Self-Care: Dedicate time each day for self-care activities that you enjoy, whether it's reading, gardening, or listening to music. Engaging in pleasurable activities can provide a valuable distraction from tinnitus.

5. Learn to Say No: Be mindful of your limits and don't hesitate to decline invitations or commitments that may exacerbate stress or fatigue. Prioritizing your well-being is crucial.

6. Maintain a Journal: Keep a journal to track your symptoms, triggers, and coping strategies. This can help identify patterns and provide insights into what works best for you.

7. Seek Professional Help When Needed: If tinnitus becomes overwhelming, consider consulting a therapist or counselor who specializes in tinnitus or chronic conditions. Professional guidance can provide valuable coping strategies.

8. Celebrate Small Wins: Acknowledge and celebrate small achievements in managing your tinnitus and maintaining balance in your life. Recognizing progress, no matter how minor, can foster a positive mindset.

Living with tinnitus involves navigating daily challenges while striving to maintain a fulfilling life. By implementing practical management strategies and finding a balance between work, social interactions, and personal well-being, individuals can improve their quality of life and develop resilience in the face of tinnitus.

CONCLUSION

Recap of Key Points

Throughout this guide, we've explored various aspects of tinnitus, from understanding its definition and types to discussing causes, symptoms, and treatment options. Key points include:

- **Understanding Tinnitus**: Tinnitus is often characterized by ringing, buzzing, or other sounds in the ears, affecting millions worldwide.
- **Types of Tinnitus**: The condition can manifest as subjective, objective, somatic, or pulsatile tinnitus, each with distinct characteristics.
- **Management Strategies**: A combination of medical treatments, sound therapy, lifestyle adjustments, and alternative therapies can help manage symptoms effectively.
- **Support Resources**: Numerous organizations, online communities,

and literature are available to provide support and information for those living with tinnitus.

Encouragement and Hope

Living with tinnitus can be challenging, but it's important to remember that you are not alone. Many individuals have found ways to manage their symptoms and lead fulfilling lives. With the right resources, support, and strategies, you can take control of your situation and reduce the impact of tinnitus on your daily life. Stay hopeful and proactive in seeking help and exploring new therapies that may arise.

As you navigate your journey with tinnitus, consider these final pieces of advice:

1. **Stay Informed**: Knowledge is empowering. Continue to educate yourself about tinnitus and stay updated on the latest research and treatment options.

2. **Be Patient**: Finding effective coping strategies may take time. Be patient with yourself as you explore what works best for you.

3. **Prioritize Self-Care**: Pay attention to your mental and physical well-being. Engage in activities that promote relaxation and joy, and don't hesitate to seek professional support when needed.

4. **Connect with Others**: Building a support network can significantly ease the emotional burden of tinnitus. Engage with communities and share your experiences.

Remember, living well with tinnitus is possible. By utilizing the strategies and resources outlined in this guide, you can work toward a balanced and fulfilling life despite the challenges tinnitus may present.

APPENDIX

Glossary of Terms

1. **Acoustic Reflex**: An involuntary muscle contraction in the middle ear that protects the inner ear from loud sounds.

2. **Cognitive Behavioral Therapy (CBT)**: A type of psychotherapy that helps individuals change negative thought patterns and behaviors related to tinnitus.

3. **Hearing Aid**: A device worn in or behind the ear that amplifies sound to assist individuals with hearing loss.

4. **Masking**: The use of background noise or sound to cover or reduce the perception of tinnitus.

5. **Neuromodulation**: A technique that alters nerve activity through electrical or magnetic stimulation, often used in tinnitus treatment.

6. **Pulsatile Tinnitus**: A type of tinnitus characterized by rhythmic sounds that often correspond to the individual's heartbeat.

7. **Sound Therapy**: A treatment approach that uses sound to reduce the perception of tinnitus and promote relaxation.

8. **Somatic Tinnitus**: A form of tinnitus that can be influenced by physical movements or changes in body position.

9. **Tinnitus Masker**: A device or tool that produces sound to mask the perception of tinnitus.

10. **Tinnitus Retraining Therapy (TRT)**: A therapeutic approach that combines sound therapy and counseling to help individuals habituate to tinnitus.

11. **Hyperacusis**: A condition where normal sounds are perceived as excessively loud or uncomfortable, often occurring alongside tinnitus.

12. **Acupuncture**: An alternative therapy involving the insertion of thin needles into specific points on the body to promote healing and relief from symptoms.

13. **Support Group**: A gathering of individuals who share similar experiences, providing emotional support and practical advice regarding tinnitus.

14. **Tinnitus Perception**: The subjective experience of hearing sounds that are not present externally, often described as ringing, buzzing, or hissing.

15. **Cochlear Implant**: A surgically implanted electronic device that bypasses damaged portions of the ear and stimulates the auditory nerve to provide a sense of sound.

This glossary serves as a reference to help readers understand key terms related to tinnitus and its management.

Frequently Asked Questions (FAQs)

1. **What is tinnitus?**
   - Tinnitus is the perception of sound, such as ringing, buzzing, or hissing, in the absence of external noise. It affects many people and can vary in intensity and type.
2. **What causes tinnitus?**
   - Common causes include hearing loss, exposure to loud noise, ear infections, certain medications, and other medical conditions. Stress and anxiety can also exacerbate symptoms.
3. **Is tinnitus a serious condition?**
   - While tinnitus itself is not usually a sign of a serious health issue, it can significantly impact quality of life. Persistent tinnitus may require evaluation and management.
4. **How is tinnitus diagnosed?**

- Diagnosis typically involves a medical history review, hearing tests, and possibly imaging studies to rule out underlying conditions. An audiologist or ear specialist usually conducts the evaluation.

5. **Can tinnitus be cured?**

   - Currently, there is no definitive cure for tinnitus, but various treatments and management strategies can help reduce its impact and improve quality of life.

6. **What treatments are available for tinnitus?**

   - Treatment options include sound therapy, cognitive behavioral therapy (CBT), medications, hearing aids, and alternative therapies such as acupuncture. Individual responses to treatment vary.

7. **How can I manage tinnitus at home?**
   - Effective home management strategies include using white noise machines, practicing relaxation techniques, maintaining a healthy lifestyle, and avoiding loud environments.

8. **Are there any dietary changes that can help?**
   - While no specific diet cures tinnitus, maintaining a balanced diet and avoiding excessive caffeine, alcohol, and salt may help some individuals manage their symptoms better.

9. **Is it normal for tinnitus to fluctuate?**
   - Yes, tinnitus can vary in intensity and perception due to factors such as stress, fatigue, exposure to noise, and overall

health. Tracking these changes can help identify triggers.

10. **Where can I find support for tinnitus?**
    - Support can be found through organizations like the American Tinnitus Association, local support groups, online forums, and social media communities where individuals share experiences and coping strategies.

www.ingramcontent.com/pod-product-compliance
Lightning Source LLC
Chambersburg PA
CBHW012257240726
48656CB00007B/2415

9798333421395